The Hypertension Cure

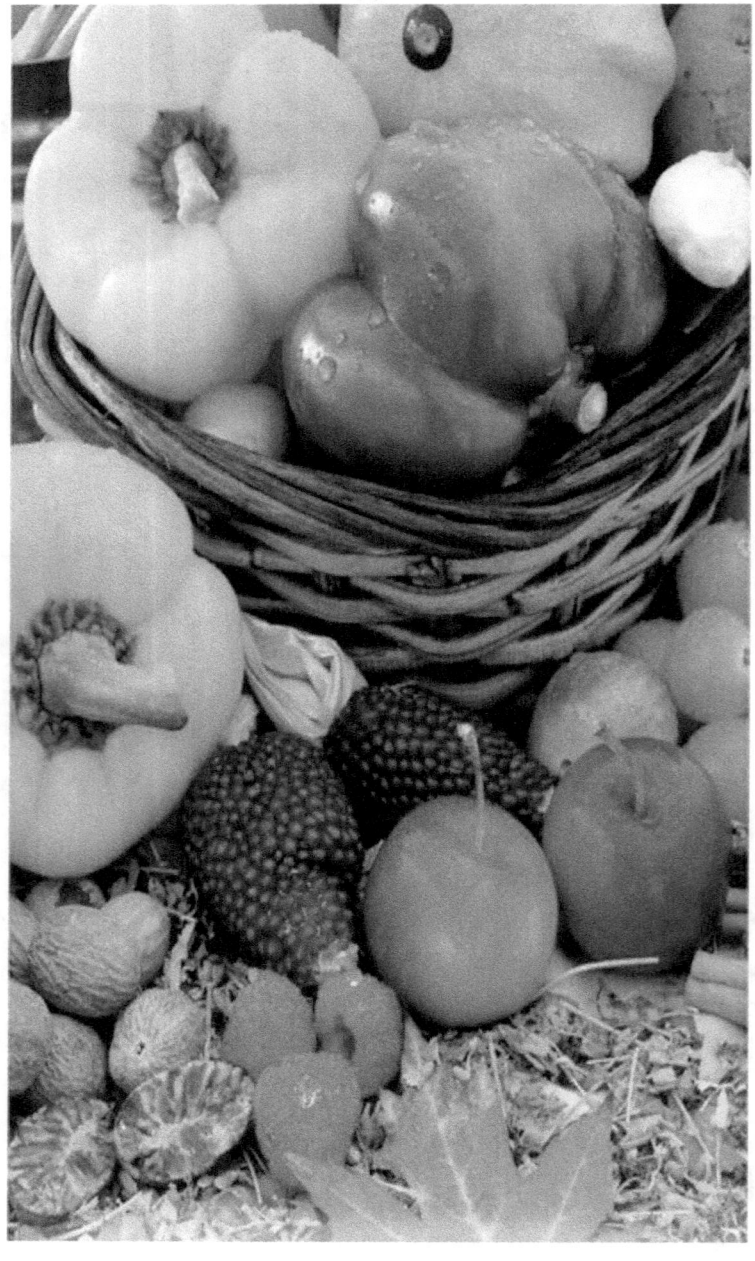

The Hypertension Cure

Lower Blood Pressure

Boost Metabolism And Get Healthy

Rossie C Pattison

The Hypertension Cure
Copyright Notice

First Printing, 2014

ISBN-13: 978-1497460843

Contents

Preface: How To Control Your Hypertension

"Watch your blood pressure!" is a warning often given in jest when something happens to irritate or excite the emotions. But high blood pressure is no joke. It can be dangerous, particularly after the middle years when hardening arteries, pushed by abnormal blood pressures beyond their capacity to expand, set the stage for sudden death or long years of invalidism.

High blood pressure the doctors call it "hypertension" is not a disease in itself. Instead, it is a symptom of various other maladies, many of them serious, others not so grave. Sometimes the causes are organic, such as diseases of the endocrine glands, the kidneys, the arteries. Frequently, however, blood pressure can be raised to an abnormally high reading by an overwrought emotional state.

But, whether the cause is organic or mental, this fact remains: High blood pressure is not a desirable condition; its cause should be ascertained, if possible, and every practicable remedy should be tested thoroughly in an effort to bring the pressure down to a safe level.

After forty-five years of age, one out of every four persons in the United States suffers from high blood pressure. Each year high blood pressure, and one of its associated diseases, hardening of the arteries, claims the lives of more than a half million Americans.

As the situation now exists, any person past the middle forties has a fifty-fifty chance of dying from apoplexy, angina pectoris, Bright's disease, coronary thrombosis all of them conditions arising from high blood pressure alone or in conjunction with hardening of the arteries.

Even more serious, it is estimated that by i960 the death toll from these two diseases hypertension and hardening of the arteries will rise to 1,200,000 victims a year, a 100 percent increase in little more than ten years!

This is a serious threat to the health of our people, a threat which should be minimized at once by a widespread educational program to warn the public of the dangers of high blood pressure, and to acquaint it with the safe remedies which have given results in hundreds of clinical trials.

If we watched our blood pressure as regularly and with as much interest as we do the gasoline or oil pressure gauges on the dashboard of our automobiles, we might avoid high blood pressure, one of the most rampant killers among the civilized diseases.

One physician, who has treated thousands of cases of high blood pressure, says that the only way to wipe out high blood pressure is for "everybody to live in the country and be poor."

What he meant is that city living and rich food cause high blood pressure to be far more prevalent among the middle and upper class urban dweller than among the poor farmer and small-town resident.

The white farmer in the southern part of the United States suffers considerably less from hypertension than his northern brother; and high blood pressure is practically unknown among the poor black tenant farmers of the South. But when the southern black man moves to an industrial center to live, his blood pressure rate went up noticeably.

The complete absence of high blood pressure among the lower classes in the hinterlands of China and Tibet, where the diet is rice and little else, has caused a flurry of "rice diet" treatments in this country on patients suffering from hypertension.

However, someone forgot to report that when these same young Chinese who lived in the "back woods" of China and ate nothing much but rice were taken from their isolated villages and put through the strain of military training and officer-training courses, they developed high blood pressure although the diet was still mainly rice!

Contrary to popular belief, blood pressure is not stable. It is as changeable as the weather. A reading taken at various intervals throughout the day would indicate widely varying fluctuations in blood pressure: the lowest being registered while the mind was calm, the body prone and at rest; the highest would occur after intense excitement, fear or anger, and after strenuous exercise.

From this it can be seen that a person with an already abnormally high blood pressure is courting suicide when he becomes excited or angry while eating a heavy meal, or while engaging in strenuous physical activity. In such an instance, he would be pushing his already high pressure up to still more dangerous heights.

And, if it so happened that the arteries had become so rigid through years of hardening that they could not accommodate the rush of this extra pressure against their brittle walls, they would rupture, bringing on a heart attack or a cerebral hemorrhage.

It is no mere figure of speech to say that "So and so will have apoplexy" when he or she learns of or experiences some disagreeable event. That, precisely, is what often happens.

The person in question is already the victim of high blood pressure; perhaps he has just eaten a heavy meal, or played a strenuous game of golf; and then he is told some extremely annoying news, or goes through some maddening experience.

Up shoots his already high blood pressure to such an elevated degree that his brittle arteries cannot withstand the extra burden. One may rupture, and he has become the victim of apoplexy, or a "stroke."

Or it might be a coronary artery that ruptures. For instance, someone with high blood pressure learns of, or witnesses, a tragic happening. The shock sends the blood pressure to such a height that a major artery in the heart breaks, bringing instant death.

Only the other day a tragic instance of this type of death was reported in the newspapers. A man in an Indiana town kissed his wife goodbye, got in the car and drove off, turning to wave to her about the time he crossed the railroad tracks that passed near their house. Apparently he did not hear the whistled warning of the oncoming train.

His car was knocked high into the air by the engine, but he was thrown clear of the wreckage, and miraculously saved from injury except for a few cuts and bruises. But back on the porch of his home, his wife had collapsed and died from an acute heart attack brought on by the horror of seeing her husband menaced, then struck, by the oncoming train.

Her heart arteries could not withstand the severe strain of a greatly increased blood pressure brought on by her extreme emotions. But sometimes it is not merely one exciting occurrence that raises the blood pressure to abnormal heights. It may be a series of con-current incidents, or an apparently intolerable situation of long duration that causes the hypertension.

Anna W. was a sensible woman, although one inclined to dramatized events out of all proportion to their true importance. When she and her husband had been married only a few years, he lost his fortune and was forced to accept a minor position in the very bank into which Anna had formerly swept, swathed in furs and sparkling with diamonds, accepting the almost servile attentions of the bank attendants.

Now she was plain Mrs. W., wife of one of the bank's employees, and not a very important one at that. On top of this blow came the humiliation of not having what she considered enough money for her personal expenditures.

It was a far cry from the $200 a week spending money and the unlimited charge accounts to the meager $15 a week now handed her to run the house and to supply her personal wants.

Although Anna loved her husband dearly and was too good a wife to complain, inwardly the situation began to take its toll of her health. It was not long before she began to suffer from palpitation of the heart and breath lessens, with pressure pains in the forehead and the back of the neck.

At first, Anna was inclined to dismiss these symptoms as of no consequence, until they became so aggravated that she was no longer able to perform her household tasks. Finally she consented to consult a doctor.

He found she had a blood pressure of "220 over 135." As we shall see later, this was a very high pressure, and certainly cause for alarm. A routine physical check-up failed to reveal the cause of her abnormal pressure. The physician wrote a prescription, told her "not to worry."

Anna went home, took the medicine faithfully and tried not to worry about herself. But, of course, this added expense of a doctor and medicine, with perhaps more such expense to come, did not alleviate her already harassed state of mind concerning money matters.

She did not get any better. The next check-up disclosed a blood pressure that had climbed a few points over the previous reading. Obviously the prior treatment had had no effect. Another drug was tried, with the same negative result.

About this time, a former friend of Anna's, a "best-selling" authoress, came to town on an autographing tour. Anna went to see her. During the course of conversation, Anna mentioned her urgent need of money.

The friend tried to press a loan on her. Anna refused, saying it was an income she wanted, not charity. After exhausting all the possibilities, it was finally decided that Anna's most likely talent was one of being able to tell an interesting story.

The authoress friend suggested that Anna devote her leisure hours to developing her writing talent, and she would endeavor to see that the stories found a market.

Months later, Anna became a selling writer, not for fabulous sums, of course, but for enough to give her the feeling of again having money of her own to spend. The blood pressure? Oh, yes, it went back to normal almost immediately after Anna's mind became so occupied with the job of becoming a successful writer that she no longer had time to brood over her reduced circumstances.

Why have I related this case history? To prove that here again, as in heart and other diseases, the mind can be the guilty one. Not only do habitual worry, fear, anxiety, anger or hatred raise the blood pressure far beyond its normal limits of fluctuation, but these continuing intense emotions also help keep the pressure up once it has been elevated.

Not everyone, however, is subject to emotionally caused hypertension. Some persons fail to show any morbid increase in blood pressure, other than a normal momentary rise, even under stress of the most intense emotions. These are usually persons of a calmer, more phlegmatic nature.

On the other hand, the average victim of mind caused high blood pressure is generally found to fit into this pattern: He tends to walk and work faster than the average; he is often more sensitive and more easily embarrassed than most persons; he does not relax often in healthful recreation; he is usually tense and irritable, with a comparatively narrow mental horizon focused with grim determination on personal aims.

Introduction

While the blood pressure of the average person may rise from only 10 to 30mm. during excitement, the person with the physical and emotional set-up conducive to high blood pressure will show a rise of from 30 to 100mm. under the same circumstances. Even though other causes of an organic nature may bring on the high blood pressure in the first place, excessive emotionalism will help keep the pressure at dangerously high levels.

An illustrative case is that of a woman who had suffered from high blood pressure for years, mainly caused by overweight and glandular disturbances arising during the menopause. But, with proper rest and diet, plus certain hormones, she was able to keep the pressure readings from reaching a dangerous level.

Then during World War II the only daughter's husband deserted her after what had appeared to be an ideal marriage, and because of religious beliefs the daughter could not sever her marital ties and begin life anew with another mate.

The mother grieved deeply because of her daughter's unhappiness and hopeless marital situation. Not long after this, the only son's new marriage also took an unhappy turn because the bride became venomously jealous of the filial attention her husband continued to pay his mother after the wedding.

The result was an ugly family scene before the honeymoon was scarcely over. The next day the mother was unable to get out of bed because of a blinding, pressing headache, a common symptom of high blood pressure.

Nor did she feel any better the next day, or the next. The family doctor was summoned barely in time to administer a sedative and avert the tragic consequences of a stroke. When he was told of the happenings that had brought on the nearly fatal rise in the mother's blood pressure, he cautioned the family to avoid all future unpleasantness and complaining, if they wanted their mother alive and out of an invalid's chair!

Of course, the more a victim of hypertension worries about his condition, living in constant dread of a heart attack or a stroke, the more his blood pressure rises.

Far better for his blood pressure, and certainly far safer for his general welfare, would it be for him to concentrate the mental energy usually spent in worry, investing his time and effort in experimenting to find a practicable remedy that would help most in his particular case. Moreover, it would be wiser for him to direct his attention toward some worthwhile project or toward developing a relaxing hobby.

Chapter 1

What Causes the Blood Pressure to Rise?

The mind has an accomplice in this "whodunit" mystery of high blood pressure. That accomplice is none other than the adrenals, two pea-sized glands that lie immediately above each kidney. Their secretion, adrenalin, is known as the "emergency hormone." It is this hormone that the mind causes the adrenals to secrete at a split second's notice in order to spur every nerve and muscle into immediate, perfectly coordinated action.

The instant that adrenalin enters the blood, the liver and spleen pour forth millions of red corpuscles into the bloodstream and the heart beats more quickly, thereby raising the blood pressure by increasing the quantity and rapidity of the flow.

And this increase is as it should be, since the adrenals were provided for that very purpose so that the body could react instantly to danger and supreme effort.

But when the mind, because of exaggerated emotions, keeps crying "Wolf, wolf!" all the time, and the adrenals keep on pouring out the "emergency hormone" into the bloodstream, the blood pressure has no way of returning to a safe, normal level.

And that is why the doctor will tell the high blood pressure sufferer, as well as the heart victim, to remain calm, to take life easy, and above all not to keep up a steady stream of nagging, worry thoughts.

The heart, as we have seen in the previous chapter, is a pump. And no pump can operate at maximum efficiency unless it is provided with a system of pipes in good condition, free from leaks and clogging corrosions.

That is the reason why any discussion of high blood pressure must also consider the human "piping system" composed of arteries, veins and capillaries.

Each of these "pipes," or blood vessels as they are rightly called, is encompassed by smooth muscle fibers arranged around the vessel. Even when the blood vessel is inactive, that is, when no great amount of blood is flowing through it at the moment, these muscle fibers continue to maintain a certain amount of tension, always on the alert to relax and contract in order to send the blood coursing through the "piping system" of the body, or to slow it down again, as the central nervous system commands.

Whenever more blood is needed, the muscle fibers relax, allowing the vascular tubes to dilate in order to accommodate the increased flow of blood. And when less blood is needed, the fibers contract, narrowing the tubes.

Notice that even the blood vessels are controlled by muscles, the same as the arms or legs. Muscles are the puppets of the body, always waiting to respond when the nervous system "jerks the strings." Like any other muscle in the body, the muscles controlling the blood vessels must be fed the proper food elements and be cleansed of waste materials to maintain them in first-class working condition. To do this is to take the most important steps toward prevention of high blood pressure.

Chapter 2

The Arteries

The arteries are the blood vessels that receive the oxygen-rich, red blood directly from the heart. They must be equipped with extremely strong walls to withstand the powerful pressure of the outwardly surging blood. Especially is this muscular strength vital in the large arteries close to the heart, such as the aorta, that great trunk artery carrying blood from the heart to the branch arteries.

The circular muscle fibers of all arteries are reinforced with alternate layers of tissue. Miraculously yet logically enough each artery has its own private system of arteries to supply these muscle tissues with nourishing blood fluid.

In addition, each arterial wall is bountifully equipped with an intricate system of nerves that regulate the diameter of the blood vessel. So please do not think of an artery as a mere rubber-like tube; it is an active organ of the body whose functioning is of prime importance to health and vigor, even to life itself. And, like any other organ of the body, the arteries can become diseased. When this happens the condition known as arteriosclerosis develops. The word means "hardening of the arteries."

Arteriosclerosis is a diagnosis any patient dreads to hear from his doctor. What it actually means is that the arterial walls are no longer flexible enough to meet the continually changing diameters that must be produced in an artery if the blood is to flow through normally in the varying quantities needed to accommodate different bodily needs.

The muscle fibers making up the arterial walls are no longer healthy enough to respond to the constant stream of commands sent out by the nervous system to "contract and relax."

The muscle fibers, through degeneration and disease, have thickened, thereby losing a large part of elasticity, a necessary characteristic since all healthy muscles must have the ability to stretch, then snap back like a piece of good rubber.

This hardening of the arteries may occur throughout the entire arterial system, or it may be confined to certain of the larger arteries such as the aorta, within the heart itself, in the brain, or in the kidneys; or it may even take place in the lower limbs, giving rise to a dangerous circulatory condition.

A healthy artery is smooth and elastic; if cut crosswise, it resembles a piece of round tubing. But when the artery begins to degenerate, here is what happens: The healthy, smooth cells on the inner wall of the artery become cloudy, then swell and die, remaining on the arterial wall as a poisonous waste.

An ulcer forms. These patches of ulcers are the actual disease of arteriosclerosis, and may often occur years before the condition known as "hardening of the arteries" makes itself known. The subsequent formations that actually harden the arteries take place either as a protective measure against the formation of more ulcers, or as a process of repair to heal the ulcers already formed.

An ulcerated artery is compared to a plastered wall that develops a crack: to repair these cracks, more plaster is spread over them, and so on every time a break occurs. Within the human body, the repair material is known as "connective tissue cells" and these cells are dispatched to all places where injuries occur. Their sole job is to replace damaged tissue.

But, like most repair work, it is only a makeshift job, efficient enough in its way, but far from approaching the perfection of the original craftsmanship. That is what takes place in any break or lesion of the tissues, when we speak of the formation of "scar tissue."

Although it has repaired and sealed the original "break" or wound, this scar tissue is bulky and thicker than the original. Within an ulcerated artery, scar tissue grows among the circular muscle walls to protect them from rupturing and springing a leak. The artery is thickened both inside and out.

Try repairing a rubber garden hose with bailing wire along most of its length, and you will have some idea of the inflexibility of the hardened, narrowed artery after scar tissue gets through with its repair job.

This is usually the type of hardened, brittle artery that many person's past middle age with hypertension often expect to withstand the constant rush of blood flowing at greatly increased pressures.

Through the compromises and makeshifts possible only with nature, the hardened arteries may be able to accommodate this high blood pressure for a long time. Then, often without warning, the arterial walls give way, and the victim suffers a heart attack or a cerebral stroke.

High blood pressure may exist without the complication of arteriosclerosis and, contrariwise, hardening of the arteries may exist without high blood pressure. But, given a combination of the two, it is almost certain that the victim will be killed by his own blood pressure, if he does not take quick, effective steps to bring the pressure down to a safer level.

The famous Dr. William Osier coined what has become almost a medical proverb when he said that "a man is as old as his arteries."

Age, although characteristically a predisposing factor in the occurrence of arteriosclerosis is not the only cause. Persons in their eighties have been examined whose arteries showed no evidence of hardening, while arteriosclerosis has been discovered in children under the age of ten.

One extreme case was that of a child only eighteen months old whose arteries were as diseased and as hardened as those found in any person of seventy.

A diagnosis of "arteriosclerosis" need not be an alarming one, for it is possible to live quite comfortably with hardened arteries —provided the blood pressure is kept at a low, safe level, and provided further that emotional upsets and strenuous activities are avoided as carefully as the plague.

Arteriosclerosis in itself, of course, can cause the blood pressure to rise, since the blood must develop greater pressure to push its way through the narrowed arteries, and a certain rise in pressure is not abnormal as one progress to an advanced age.

But this is all the more reason why all other factors that would contribute to high blood pressure must be located and eliminated, if the blood pressure is not to be raised to dangerously high levels.

Hardening of the arteries, however, is but one of the disease conditions associated with high blood pressure. Another common cause is overweight, especially when it reaches the morbid stage known as obesity.

An overweight person, otherwise healthy, will have a blood pressure that averages some 9 mm. higher than normal. And a person actually obese will show an even greater rise in pressure.

The obvious cure for high blood pressure brought on by overweight is to get rid of the extra pounds of fat. A person with blood pressure as high as 160 to 170 can always reduce the reading to normal simply by reducing the weight of his body to the proper figure.

There is sufficient evidence against certain of the endocrine glands to warrant suspecting them in the sudden onset of hypertension. Especially do the adrenal, the pituitary and the thyroid glands come under suspicion in this connection.

In cases of this type, the glandular system is found to be overactive. Extracts that regulate the endocrine glandular system are usually found to be effective in lowering this type of hypertension. For many years it has been suspected that the kidneys had some-thing to do with causing high blood pressure. An acute kidney inflammation that only temporarily puts the kidneys out of good working order will not influence the blood pressure to any great degree.

But chronic kidney diseases that last for months and years will, in the long run, bring about high blood pressure in most patients.

The most permanent type of high blood pressure yet produced in the research laboratories has been that resulting from damaged kidneys. When the kidneys are normal, they secrete two substances called renin and anti-renin in proportions that balance each other.

An injured or diseased kidney, however, will secrete more renin, and it is this excess of renin that so often causes permanently high blood pressure. When speaking of an "injured" or a "diseased" kidney, I do not necessarily mean that the high blood pressure will show up the next day, or even within the year after the kidneys become damaged.

But in hundreds of cases where high blood pressure has put in an unexplained appearance, and remained despite all efforts to lower it, an investigation into the medical history of the patient has revealed that in the past the patient experienced a slight kidney disturbance; possibly a trace of albumin in the urine was the only symptom, one which the doctor advised his patient not to become unduly alarmed about.

So the patient did nothing to correct an obviously abnormal condition; then, years later, high blood pressure with all its ominous possibilities put in its appearance.

Or perhaps the kidneys had been left in a weakened condition after some childhood ailment such as measles, scarlet fever, diphtheria, even tonsillitis. It might even have been a serious bout with pneumonia that affected the kidneys so they would secrete too much renin.

Even more likely, the kidney damage may have been caused by some of the dangerous drugs that have been prescribed during recent years in such copious quantities (often merely as an experiment).

I refer specifically to the sulfa drugs whose disastrous effect on the kidneys will be admitted by every honest medical man.

There are many case histories where treatment of the diseased kidneys also cleared up high blood pressure in a patient after all other efforts to lower the pressure had failed. An illustration in point is that of a Boston attorney whose case came to my attention during one of my lectures in that city.

The man's daughter mentioned to me that her father was becoming more unequal each day to the effort of carrying on his profession because of the physical toll that the symptoms of his high blood pressure (throbbing headaches, extreme fatigue and dizziness) were exacting from his reserve energy. He was on the verge of a nervous collapse from the strain.

After questioning the daughter closely about her father's medical history, I learned that he had been in a train wreck some years before, suffering a kidney injury so serious that for a while the doctors thought it would have to be removed.

However this extreme measure proved unnecessary, and the patient apparently made a complete recovery. Yet the aftermath of this kidney injury was the high blood pressure that was now incapacitating this attorney.

I suggested that the man's hypertension be treated by making an effort to restore his kidneys to as nearly normal functioning as possible. This was done, and I learned later that all the more annoying symptoms of his hypertension had disappeared.

The "rice diet" for high blood pressure has received a lot of publicity recently and I feel it my duty to include some mention of it, if only because it might possibly bring relief to some sufferer who had tried all other sensible remedies and still failed to get relief from hypertension.

The rice diet is claimed to have given at least temporary relief to some hypertensive patients, while others received absolutely no benefits. But I must emphasize that I do not recommend the rice diet, if only because it is too low in protein, that most essential of all food elements.

However, if anyone insists on trying the rice diet as a cure for high blood pressure, they would be well advised to offset this lack of vitally needed protein by taking amino acids in concentrated form.

In this way only can symptoms of protein deficiency be prevented from developing in a body already harassed with high blood pressure. I realize it is claimed with good reason that high blood pressure is not prevalent in China among those whose chief item of diet is rice.

And yet, on the other hand, all the symptoms of protein deficiency muscular weakness, lassitude, swollen limbs, and poor mental capacity are widespread among these same Chinese who do not suffer from high blood pressure.

And so with a rice diet, it seems to be a case of making up one's mind which evil is preferable high blood pressure, or protein-deficiency diseases.

Even the doctors who have prescribed the rice diet will admit they do not know why it works, when it does. It is not improbable to reason that in the cases where this almost starvation diet worked, it was because of the weight lost that the patient's blood pressure dropped.

Chapter 3

Removing Certain Foods from your Diet

Removing all rich foods and limiting the diet to moderate portions of proteins such as meat, fish, chicken and cheese (supplemented by concentrated amino acids) plus raw and cooked low-starch fruits and vegetables would no doubt have accomplished the same good results. A mere reduction in the consumption of fatty foods to the absolute minimum will work wonders with one type of arteriosclerosis caused by fatty degeneration of the arterial walls, called atherosclerosis.

This type of arterial disease is rare among the Chinese and the Okinawans who get little or no fat in their diets. During and after the First World War when the fat shortage became acute in Germany, doctors in that country noticed that atherosclerosis decreased to a marked degree.

Further, this type of hardened arteries is rarely found in persons who are chronic alcoholics, simply because a heavy drinker is seldom a heavy consumer of fatty foods.

Therefore, it would be my personal theory that the rice diet works for some victims of hypertension and not for others because those benefited are persons suffering from this type of hardening of the arteries.

The stringent rice diet restricts their consumption of fatty foods to the point where the arterial condition improves, thereby alleviating the hypertension. The same effect might just as well be obtained with a diet still containing a negligible quantity of fats, and yet including adequate portions of necessary protein.

It might be well to mention one other dietary factor that is suspected of contributing to arteriosclerosis, and thereby to high blood pressure, and that is cholesterol, a fatty substance found in large amounts in egg yolk, cream, brains, sweetbreads, oysters, fish roe, animal fats and chocolate.

Although there is no clinical proof as yet that eating foods containing large amounts of cholesterol will cause heart and blood vessel diseases in humans, still we do know that arteriosclerosis has been produced in rabbits and chickens by feeding them an excess quantity of this fatty substance.

That is why the suggestion is made that persons with a tendency toward high blood pressure and heart disease arising from hardened coronary arteries, as well as those definitely the victims of arterial degeneration, would do well to exclude the above high cholesterol items from their diet, and to eat sparingly of all other fatty foods.

Foods eaten by the high blood pressure patient should also be low in starches and sugar, with absolutely no spices or condiments. Four or five light meals a day are far better than three heavy meals.

In fact, the obese patient will have to put himself on a sensible reducing diet containing plenty of protein and low starch fruits and vegetables, preferably eaten raw. Ample water should be taken between meals to keep the kidneys well flushed, thereby avoiding damage to these delicate organs.

No longer is it considered wise to remove meat from the diet of the high blood pressure patient. In fact, the protein contained in lean beef and lamb (pork has too much fat to be included in the diet of the hypertensive patient) is needed to help repair any muscle damage caused in the arterial walls by the excessive blood pressure.

Often it is advisable to supplement the diet with extra proteins in the form of easily assimilated amino acids to assure plenty of muscle-repairing material in the body at all times, in the event the stomach is not capable of fully digesting meat protein.

Very little or no salt should be used, especially when there is the complicating factor of hardening arteries. And certainly no one was ever the worse for using a minimum of common table salt.

Nature provided all the salt we need in the form of other compounds contained naturally in meats, fruits, grains, vegetables and dairy products. No salt is the best rule for the person afflicted with high blood pressure.

Chapter 4

Dieting and Weight loss

Keep it moderate, balanced and sensible is my final admonition. There are dietary supplements which admittedly have brought immeasurable relief from high blood pressure. The vitamin niacin, found in the B-complex group, is particularly effective in preventing and relieving the type of high blood pressure that is linked to nerves and nervousness.

When the nerves of the heart and blood vessels suffer from a niacin deficiency, they tend to make these organs taut, thus bringing on a rise in blood pressure. As a specific remedy for high blood pressure of this type, it is often advisable to supplement the diet with either vitamin B complex or niacin concentrate in tablet form.

Vitamin B-complex itself is also recommended by Dr. L. Calder as a preventive for high blood pressure. Containing the nerve vitamins thiamin and niacin, B-complex will help control the type of high blood pressure arising from nervous excitability.

Two other vitamins, A and P, help control high blood pressure. Vitamin P, present in citrus juice, especially lemon, acts to maintain the small capillaries in good condition, preventing their breaking down and bleeding into the tissues. Injury of this kind to the small blood vessels in the kidneys is one type of renal damage that is a direct cause of high blood pressure.

Vitamin A is also necessary for proper functioning of the inner lining of the kidney tubules, helping to keep the kidneys healthy and functioning properly, thus avoiding the secretion of excessive renin, the substance that sends the blood pressure skyrocketing when too much of it gets into the bloodstream.

In connection with keeping the kidneys healthy as a means of preventing high blood pressure, I should also mention the herb fenugreek.

Numerous case histories attest the efficacy of this herb, brewed into a tea, as a cleansing, soothing agent for the kidneys, helping them prevent poisonous accumulations that bring on disease and degeneration of the renal tissues.

Also, the herb fenu greek contains choline, a lipotropic (fat-dissolving) substance that is being used clinically in an effort to dissolve the deposits of fat (cholesterol) that accumulate on the arterial walls, causing these blood vessels to lose their elasticity and to harden.

There is still another natural remedy for high blood pressure which has met with a high degree of success, although certain medical opinion is as skeptical of its efficacy as I am of the so-called "rice diet."

This remedy for high blood pressure is nothing more complex, or more dangerous, than the well-known herb garlic, combined with watercress and parsley.

European medical men have long contended that the results obtained with garlic as a treatment for high blood pressure were worthwhile, while American doctors have dismissed the idea.

But then, European medicine always did lean more toward natural herbal remedies, while our doctors placed most of their faith in the powerful, synthetic drugs.

For some reason not exactly clear, garlic as a remedy for high blood pressure works much more effectively when combined with watercress.

One herb seems to complement the other, whether taken in tablet form or used as salad ingredients.

The garlic and the watercress, then, are the therapeutic agents in garlic tablets, while parsley is included to reduce the objectionable odor of the garlic. In other words, parsley makes the garlic "more sociable."

The action of garlic in treating high blood pressure is readily explained. This herb has proved its worth in hundreds of cases of hypertension because it eases the spasms of the small arteries, thus reducing the pressure and tension that are characteristic symptoms of this disease.

Clinical research has proved that in some cases the administration of garlic to a hypertensive patient actually lessened the tension within the arteries.

Chapter 5

Healing Garlic

Garlic also slows the pulse and helps modify the heart rhythm, at the same time often relieving the annoying symptoms such as dizziness, numbness, breathless-ness and insomnia. Let me stress that garlic is not a cure for high blood pressure. Its sole action is to relieve and lessen the painful, dangerous symptoms of this disease which in itself is nothing but a symptom of another disorder elsewhere in the body.

However, it has been noted in many cases that the continued use of garlic has tended to bring excessive blood pressures down to a permanently safe level.

As for garlic not being a cure for high blood pressure, medical men will admit that they wished they were as certain of the cure for high blood pressure as they were of some of its causes.

Each treatment is nothing but an experiment; what works with one patient may fail with another suffering from high blood pressure arising from substantially the same cause.

In treating disorder arising from as complicated a mechanism as the human organic system, there is only one safe thing to assume: That every treatment should be in the nature of an experiment and that the experiment should be performed with substances of natural origin which will leave the patient with no harmful aftereffects such as often occur from the use of strong drugs.

Even the doctors are agreed that few drugs will help high blood pressure. And even the one or two that do contribute a little relief are so dangerous in large amounts that their use is necessarily limited.

The best way to attack high blood pressure, even the persistent type caused by diseased kidneys, is through diet and dietary supplements. Proper meals and vitamin and herbal supplements are sane remedies.

Frequently not only do they relieve the high blood pressure but they also add immeasurably to general health. As an added precaution, the high blood pressure patient must get at least eight hours of sleep and relaxation each night, as well as finding time to relax during the day, preferably after lunch, if possible. Drink plenty of water to keep the kidneys well flushed, avoid constipation and learn to control the emotions. High blood pressure can be a killer, but it can also be so managed that its victim is allowed to live out and enjoy his allotted span of years.

Chapter 6

The Gall Bladder and Liver

BILE, the product of the liver, can actually "color" your personality. When the gall bladder, that pear-shaped, bile storage sac hanging from the underside of the liver, kicks up a disturbance, the result is more than physical, since bile makes itself felt mentally as well. This matter of bile can also be a two way trouble track, since our state of mind has a great deal to do with the manufacture and flow of bile and too much or too little bile emptying from the gall bladder can mean a changed personality!

In fully 80 percent of the cases, gall bladder disease and gallstones are believed to be related to nervous or emotional upsets.

Case history after case history emphasizes the fact that attacks of gall bladder trouble come on after a family row, extreme mental depression, marital unhappiness, money worries, or just plain worries for the sake of giving the mind some negative exercise.

So closely related are a patient's disposition and his gall bladder and liver; that sometimes a diagnosis can be made merely by observing his temper.

The next time anyone brushes rudely past you on the bus, or in the store, muttering uncomplimentary things about you for being in his or her way, look closely at that person's face.

More likely than not, you will see a yellow, "bilious-looking" skin, tightly compressed lips, muddy whites of the eyes, as well as hands dotted with dark brown spots like large freckles. And, if you are unfortunate enough to come close, you will notice a very unpleasant breath.

All these symptoms are characteristic of a poorly functioning gall bladder and liver. It is not clairvoyance to be able to predict that anyone who is easily irritated and who exhibits violent dislikes toward others, even strangers, is the victim of too much or too little bile.

How often we have heard the expression: "He surely looks at things with a jaundiced eye." The liver, where bile is manufactured, is more greatly influenced by the emotions than any other of the digestive organs. A feeling of joy and contentment causes a normal, moderate amount of bile to flow into the gall bladder, ready to be poured into the upper intestine where fats are finally broken down.

This is the real reason why too much emphasis cannot be placed on the fact that mealtime is not the time to hash over old wrongs, to discuss the family budget or to upbraid Junior for his poor scholastic showing. Man's digestive apparatus was designed to function best under cheerful, relaxed conditions.

Sorrow causes far more bile to flow into the gall bladder than can be used, thereby setting the stage for the formation of those troublesome little rock crystals called gallstones. The habit of gloom or self-pity brings on real trouble by way of the liver and the gall bladder.

Anger stops the flow of bile almost completely. The man who takes part in a heated argument while eating a meal of fried steak, french-fried potatoes and pie is going to suffer worse indigestion than the man who remains calm while eating these unwise viands.

Why? Because the calm man's gall bladder will probably provide enough bile to break down these fatty foods into at least half-way digestible form; but the angry man's gall bladder will be as empty of bile as though it had been drained, all because the liver was affected by his heated emotions.

A strong feeling of loathing or nausea while eating will cause the entire biliary system to contract; this includes the small bile channels in the liver, the gall bladder and the duct that carries bile to the intestine.

This sudden squeezing shut of the gall bladder dams up the bile, and if the pressure becomes too great, bile may be forced into the heart and blood vessels. When this occurs, the miserable condition known as jaundice sets in.

Jaundice may also occur in any person regardless of the mental attitude when the small intestine and the bile passages become afflicted by catarrh. This is an inflammatory condition that causes these parts to become clogged with stagnant mucus.

Treatment for jaundice always aims at clearing out the bile passages so the bile can flow freely again in the intended direction instead of remaining dammed up in the liver where it oozes out into the bloodstream to be distributed throughout the body cells. This is what causes the characteristically yellowish skin and eyeballs of a jaundiced person.

Chapter 7

Gall Bladder

Bile, or gall as it is commonly known, is a golden yellow fluid so acrid that "bitter as gall" has become a cliché. This digestive juice stimulates the pancreas into contributing its digestive ferments to the process of digestion; it also emulsifies fat foods, that is, reduces them to a liquid. Bile does this job by dividing the large food fat particles into very fine droplets. When digestion is normal, all fatty food is turned into "milk" in the duodenum by the bile that pours into it from the gall bladder.

Unless fats are readily converted into this milk, the body can absorb only minute traces of fat, and this interferes with the proper balance in the body between the proteins, carbohydrates and fats. One common symptom of poor fat digestion is a never-satisfied appetite.

Bile is the body's own laxative substance; it stimulates peristalsis, that wave-like action keeping intestinal contents on the move. A third very vital function of bile has been established quite recently. Without proper quantities of bile present in the duodenum during the digestive process, vitamins A, D and K cannot properly be absorbed from the food eaten.

If sufficient bile is not sent by the sensitive gall bladder nerves into the intestines, these vitamins are passed from the body in the waste matter instead of being absorbed by the bloodstream.

For this reason, if for no other, disorders of the liver or gall bladder should not go on unchecked; the nagging, uncomfortable symptoms of gall bladder upsets or even the acute pains resulting from an obstructed bile duct are but half the evil.

More insidious is the general breakdown in health occasioned by prolonged cell starvation when not enough vitamins A, D and K reach the bloodstream through the intestinal walls because insufficient bile has interfered with the assimilation of these food elements.

A healthy gall bladder should empty itself of bile almost completely two or three times every 24 hours. This emptying in a normal gall bladder is caused by regular rhythmic contractions of the sac.

But so delicate is the nerve poise of this small organ that almost anything may upset its emptying rhythm fear, excitement, grief, worry, fatigue, certain drugs, too much of the wrong kind of food. Any or all of these conditions may cause the gall bladder to stop the regular contractions that force the bile out into the duct leading to the upper intestine.

A diet too high in fats overworks the gall bladder, while a diet devoid of fats allows complete stagnation of the bile within the gall bladder. Both types of diet are unwise. An effort should be made to strike the happy fat medium that will give the gall bladder a chance to perform as nature intended.

A small amount of fat should be taken with the food, especially on reducing diets; to keep the gall bladder stimulated enough to empty itself.

From the days of ancient Rome, olive oil has been a safe, popular remedy for persons suffering from disorders of the gall bladder. Olive oil, although it will not cure the disorder, will make it easier for the gall bladder to send bile into the intestines instead of harboring it within the bladder itself and the bile duct.

About two tea spoonful of a good, pure olive oil taken every day either plain or mixed with the food is a wise addition to any diet. However, I do not recommend salad oils made from cotton seed; these have been known to produce chronic digestive upsets, particularly colitis, in many persons.

Bile is a fluid composed chiefly of bile salts, bile pigments (the greenish brown chemicals that give the characteristic yellow coloring), lecithin and cholesterol. This last ingredient is the real troublemaker, causing the formation of gallstones. Cholesterol is the bile substance that forms the sediment from which stones gradually crystallize.

The hard, crusty substances found caked in water pipes and tea kettles, especially in hard water regions, offer a good comparison for what happens when bile is allowed to back up in the gall bladder over a long period of time.

Cholesterol

Little masses of cholesterol are precipitated from the bile and remain in the gall bladder. This cholesterol sediment, once formed, is never dissolved. From this solid precipitation the gallstones grow, starting out as one single crystal, attaching itself to another crystal, becoming larger and larger until the stones range in size all the way from a pinhead to that of a marble.

Extreme cases have been observed where the stone even reached the size of a hen's egg. A stone, once it starts to form, is like a snowball rolling down hill; more and more of the cholesterol sediment will attach itself to the stones already formed.

Gallstones resemble agates in chemical structure and physical appearance. A stone that has been removed from the body is a beautiful iridescent ochre yellow or a shining malachite green, far prettier than some of the semi-precious stones with which women adorn themselves.

Naturally this beauty cannot be appreciated by anyone who has experienced the excruciating pain of a gallstone trying to pass through the narrow bile duct!

About 25 percent of all adults harbor gallstones at least those living under civilized eating conditions. At the age of twenty, one person in a 100 has gallstones; at fifty years of age, 1 in 10, and at sixty-five years, 1 in 5 persons will be found to have stones present in the gall bladder.

Oddly enough, diseases of the gall bladder, especially stones, are more frequent in women than in men. Particularly is this true in stout women over the age of forty who have had at least one or two pregnancies.

The crowding and gorging of the gall bladder that takes place during pregnancy is thought to account for the high incidence of gall bladder disorders among women who have had children.

But these "fair, fat and forty" women also have two strikes against them, regardless of whether or not they have ever been pregnant: First, they probably have acquired their plumpness through overindulgence in rich foods; and second, they perhaps have gained the weight rapidly, having resigned themselves to the joys of the dinner table in compensation for lost romance.

Also, they may bring on an attack of gallstones by trying to get rid of that excess weight as rapidly as they gained it! Any, or all, of these conditions predispose toward gall bladder disorders.

Not everyone with gallstones, however, suffers because of their presence in the gall bladder. It is only when a stone gets restless and starts to move that it may if too large block the narrow bile duct that connects the gall bladder with the upper intestine. When this happens, the spasms of pain are violent. One medical man has de-scribed the pain of gallstone colic as equaling the severity of childbirth pains.

At first, the symptoms of gallstones are vague and hard to diagnose. It is only when an attack on gallstone colic occurs that their presence can be diagnosed for certain.

Hundreds of tiny stones may form within the gall bladder before one grows large enough to block the bile duct. A person may carry around a load of gallstones, like marbles in a sack, for years without feeling any pain.

But such a person is like Damocles of mythological fame who was compelled to dine sitting under a sword that hung by a single hair, never knowing when the hair would break and the sword strike him.

The presence of stones in the gall bladder is sufficient cause for an attack of gallstone colic. Sometimes the stones give a "preview" performance by causing pain and tenderness in the right side of the abdomen, especially around the ninth rib and under the right shoulder blade. When this happens, the victim often diagnoses it as "liver trouble" or "indigestion pains."

Pain or tenderness in the regions mentioned above should be reason enough for caution about the diet. But when these symptoms are coupled with chronic constipation, heartburn, gas pains, belching, bloating, nausea, loss of appetite, bad breath and stubborn headaches, the time has come for immediate action, if more serious consequences are to be averted. Any one or more of these symptoms ordinarily point directly at the gall bladder.

A case of mistaken diagnosis was brought to my attention not too long ago. A middle-aged man had complained of a pressure headache that seemed to encircle his head. Also his vision had become noticeably poorer since the onset of the headaches.

Half way through a line of print his eyes would seem to jump a line or two, and it would take some effort on his part to re-focus them properly. A change in eyeglasses did not correct the trouble. Then the headaches became so severe that he was no longer able to work.

The physician called in on the case suspected a brain tumor, and he held a consultation with two brain specialists. The consensus was that the headache and the disturbance in vision were being caused by a tumor on the brain. Surgery, they agreed, was risky but the only answer.

The man's daughter, however, was not satisfied with the diagnosis. She prevailed upon another doctor, who happened to be an osteopath as well as an expert diagnostician, to look at her father. When this doctor entered the sick room, his immediate thought was,

"This is a case of an upset gall bladder, judging by the smell of the patient's breath." He examined the sick man, asked him a few questions, and gave his diagnosis as a poorly functioning gall bladder.

The other physicians scoffed at this opinion and insisted upon the operation. However, the daughter was adamant that her father give the last doctor a chance to clear up his headache before submitting to highly dangerous brain surgery.

Within three weeks the man was back on the job, his headaches gone, and his digestion better than in years, his eyesight improved 100 percent! The gall bladder had been the source of all his misery.

After it had been stimulated into getting rid of its backed-up bile, the symptoms of the "brain tumor" disappeared. A diseased gall bladder may be the result of infection, and may occur without involving the formation of stones. Such an infection can come from invasions of bacteria draining into the system from infected teeth, sinuses or from a pus-laden appendix.

Typhoid fever often leaves its victims with bacteria, whole colonies of which make their way to the gall bladder where they take up permanent residence, later causing infections and inflammations.

Although inflammation or infection of the gall bladder may take place without gallstones having formed, a gall bladder that is allowed to remain chronically inflamed or infected paves the way for stone formations.

Chapter 8

Vitamin A

Large daily doses of vitamin A (upwards of 1,000 units), together with at least 300 milligrams of choline, may prevent the formation of gallstones. This combination seems to make the gall bladder work more normally, preventing its becoming sluggish. And to supplement the good work of vitamin A and choline within the gall bladder, vitamin C is also helpful, together with sufficient daily quantities of the organic minerals iron, chlorine, magnesium, potassium and sodium.

These vitamin and mineral elements seem to provide the favorable chemical background for secretion of the hormone cholecystokinin whose job it is to open the valve of the bile duct so that bile can flow freely instead of remaining dammed up within the duct and stagnating within the gall bladder.

Proper eating habits, of course, are of prime importance for anyone disposed to gall bladder disorders. To build your meals around rich viands and fried foods fried steak and potatoes, pies and rich desserts is to stick out your neck and ask for gall bladder trouble.

Alcohol is another reason why the gall bladder often does not work the way it should. Anyone who has experienced enough warning twinges to make him suspect trouble in the gall bladder would do well to adopt a diet consisting of plain, simple foods.

Since cholesterol is the material of which gallstones are formed, it is wise to avoid the foods that contain a too high content of this fatty substance, such as egg yolk, caviar, sweetbreads, liver, kidneys and animal fat.

It is also important to exclude from the diet all condiments and spices, all fried and fatty foods (except olive oil and butter) and coarse, fibrous vegetables. Gas-forming foods, especially onions and members of the cabbage family, are likely to stir up trouble.

Foods allowed on a diet for gall bladder disorders are: Lean meat (except pork), shrimps, oysters, cottage cheese made from skimmed milk, low-fat fish (but no canned salmon or sardines), chopped vegetables (except those with tough fibers, and tomatoes, unless strained of the seeds), fruit juices, cooked fruits containing no seeds, cooked cereals, gelatins and jellies.

If giving up tea or coffee would be a real hardship, it may be taken, but only after being greatly weakened with hot water. Strictly taboo are rich gravies and sauces, cream soups, ice cream, alcohol, carbonated drinks, vinegar and pepper. In fact, these last two items might well be excluded from the kitchen altogether in the interest of better digestion for everyone.

A glass of grapefruit or orange juice taken before breakfast and a tea made from fenugreek herb before retiring have proved good additions to the health regimen of those who must adhere to a strict diet.

The citrus juice promotes the proper degree of acidity in the stomach so that maximum digestion of proteins can take place, while the herb tea acts as a soothing and cleansing agent throughout the digestive tract.

Plenty of water should be drunk throughout the day to keep the bile tract well supplied with enough liquid to prevent its becoming overly concentrated. Smaller, more frequent meals are preferable to three heavy meals.

Breakfast should be ample enough to cause the gall bladder to give up the large flow of bile that has accumulated in it during the night. A "tea and toast" breakfast is a foolish habit.

A gall bladder that has gotten out of line, or one that threatens to kick up trouble, can be lived with if common sense is made the keynote of the daily regimen. It is also well to remember that a moderate amount of physical exercise, together with deep breathing, is an excellent stimulant for the gall bladder.

A Chicago executive who was plagued with gall bladder trouble was forced to take a six months' rest in the country because of a nervous breakdown.

All the while he was following the simple, restful routine of outdoor living, coupled with ample physical exercise; he was able to forget that he ever had such a thing as a gall bladder.

Yet as soon as he returned to the tense, sedentary life that his position demanded, he began to feel the old familiar twinges again.

Moderation in eating plus deep breathing, plenty of water, at least eight hours' rest, calm attitude (particularly at mealtime), and the addition of vitamins A and C, choline and organic minerals in concentrated form as a dietary supplement are the best prescription for the gall bladder sufferer.

Chapter 9

Liver

Talking about the gall bladder before the liver is rather like reading the end of a story first, since it is the liver that manufactures the bile stored in the gall bladder. The liver is the factory, while the gall bladder is merely the supply depot. But because the liver is all too often blamed for common troubles that arise in the gall bladder, I preferred discussing the real culprit first.

The average liver in the human body will weigh close to three pounds, and it occupies the entire space under the right half of the diaphragm. It is the largest gland in the body, being a blood-filled sponge through which must flow every drop of blood returning from the intestines to the heart.

Within this sponge-like organ the filtered blood flows upward toward the heart, while a parallel stream of newly manufactured bile flows downward toward the gall bladder. The liver is "man's best friend," for it saves his life many times daily. This is true because the liver acts as a filter between the intestines and the heart. Poisonous substances often sneak past the intestinal walls.

Without the liver, these toxins would paralyze the heart function almost instantly. Poisons such as nicotine, caffeine, morphine and atropine go through a chemical reaction in the liver that transforms them into harmless compounds.

A small dose of atropine, for example, injected directly into the veins of an animal will cause death; yet four times the same dose may be injected into the portal vein leading from the intestines into the liver, and the animal will remain alive.

The reason is that the liver removes the poison from the drug before allowing it to enter the hepatic vein that leads out of the liver toward the heart. Germs, too, as well as broken-down red blood cells, are taken out of the blood and literally eaten by the liver cells.

It is within the liver that amino acids are rebuilt into proteins that feed human cells science has estimated that about 1,600 different human proteins are supplied by the liver from different combinations of the 23 amino acids.

Digestion in intestines has previously broken down food protein into these amino acids from which the liver reconstructs human protein. In recent years it has also been discovered that the liver is responsible for activating the hormone insulin secreted by the pancreas to burn sugar in the body cells. Doctors have observed numerous cases of diabetes that developed even when the pancreas was healthy and supplying adequate insulin to the bloodstream.

The trouble in these cases was traced to the liver. This organ was found to be faulty or so badly diseased that it could not activate the insulin secreted by a healthy pancreas, thereby leaving the body in the same fix as that of a true diabetic condition that could not manufacture its own insulin supply and had to depend upon injections of this hormone.

In many of these cases, normal metabolism of sugar was restored in the patient merely by treating and overcoming the defect in the liver. In view of the liver's varied and highly important functions, human health demands that the liver be kept in good working condition at all times. This vital organ must not be allowed to become diseased or to break down under the strain of overwork.

Even though the liver has the power to render most poisons harmless, it is well to remember that even the most faithful bodyguard will eventually break down under the strain of being called upon too frequently for rescue work. Heavy coffee, tea and alcohol drinkers, as well as tobacco smokers, can push the liver too far with excessive amounts of these drugs to render harmless every day.

Also, because the liver is built to act as a dam for all fluids, an excessive intake of liquid, over a long period of time, especially alcoholic drinks such as beer, may cause the liver to become as hard as a board. This is called cirrhosis of the liver.

As a further duty, the liver must store emergency quantities of glycogen, the energy sugar in a stable form. If extra amounts of body sugar (and by "sugar" I do not mean the atrocity we know as white beet or cane sugar) are needed by the muscles to carry the body through strenuous physical activities, the liver, like a provident storekeeper, has it on hand to dispatch promptly.

Moreover, the liver is the "vitamin and mineral shop" of the body. It extracts from carrots and other vegetables that substance; carotene which has proved a valuable food element in maintaining healthy eyes.

But carotene, as it exists in the vegetable juices, cannot be utilized by the body, because first it must be converted into vitamin A. And that is where the liver enters the scene, extracting vitamin A from carotene and storing it for future use within the body. In addition, the liver collects and stores all members of the vitamin B-complex group, as well as vitamins C and D.

In the liver are also stored iron and copper, both so urgently needed before the bone marrow can produce the healthy red blood cells that prevent anemia.

To produce prothrombin, a substance without which even the tiniest cut would prove fatal, the liver extracts vitamin K from our food; this gives normal blood the ability to clot.

A damaged, badly operating liver can be suspected when there is frequent bleeding from the nose or from hemorrhoids. A serious bodily infection that has overworked the liver by sending a lot of toxic substances into the body will also cause this excessive bleeding from the nose or the rectum.

What this temporary bleeding symptom usually means is that the liver is not able to extract vitamin K and produce prothrombin in normal amounts.

Red blood cells cannot be formed within the bone marrow until the liver first supplies it with what is called the "anti-anemia factor." An infection of long standing, such as that which often hides away in the sinuses, will so weaken the liver that anemia sets in because not enough of this anti-anemia factor can be provided.

Anemia patients should seek to determine whether their blood deficiency is the result of inadequate iron in the diet, or whether the situation is further complicated by a long-established infection somewhere in the body.

If only we could realize what often irreparable damage we do to the most versatile organ in our body by compelling it to handle needless quantities of poisons, I am sure most of us would be a little more considerate of our liver.

It merits the respect and loving care given a rich uncle. How I wish I could get the sleeping pill addicts, as well as the habitual users of strong medicines and drugs, to realize what they are doing to one of the most vital organs in their body.

After great quantities of the poisons contained in alcohol and in every drug are taken into the body, the liver, which has stepped forth nobly to assimilate these excessive toxins in order to spare the heart, is so strained from overwork that it becomes "sluggish."

No longer can it work at normal efficiency to produce the proteins, vitamins and minerals that are food for our body cells; nor can it manufacture bile in sufficient quantities to assure maximum digestion of fats. Even small doses of aspirin, a potentially dangerous drug, taken regularly will eventually harm the liver.

Since the liver is a "wise" organ that tries to protect foolhardy man against the abuse he heaps upon his own digestive tract, the greater portion of our civilized diseases originate because of an overworked, damaged liver.

The majority of persons nearing forty have livers working at considerably less than par, because of years devoted to too much of the wrong kind of food. Excess fats, starches and sweets are a direct cause of liver breakdown.

When the excessive use of these foods is coupled with inadequate protein foods, as so frequently is the case, the liver is harmed even more because it does not have an adequate supply of the amino acids from which to reconstruct the human protein that its own cells, as well as others throughout the body, must have to keep from dying from starvation.

In addition to a perfect balance of all amino acids, any diet under-taken to prevent or relieve a disordered liver should include these vitamins in at least the daily quantities indicated: vitamin A, 25,000 units; vitamin B-1 (thiamin), 10 milligrams; riboflavin, 5 milligrams; vitamin C, 2,000 units.

Vitamin E also should be included, although the daily quantities needed have not as yet been definitely established. If the foods available for the diet cannot supply all these vitamins in at least the quantities indicated, it might be an extra health safeguard to rely upon vitamin concentrates to supplement a diet deficient in these food elements.

Amino acids, especially, are needed in ample quantity to avoid liver damage, since it has been proved that the human protein made from these "protein building blocks" and stored in the liver also protects the liver cells themselves from harmful, toxic substances. In an earlier chapter we have seen that the liver has first call on all the glutamic acid (one of the 23 aminos) taken into the body.

If any is left over after the liver has supplied its needs, the brain gets what remains in the bloodstream. Anyone who wishes maximum brain health, as well as liver efficiency, must surely provide enough glutamic acid in the diet to keep both these organs well supplied with this food element which seems to be so vital to their wellbeing.

A lack of protein in the diet is one way to invite trouble in this "king of organs," the liver. Vegetarians, and older persons whose teeth or digestive organs cannot handle large enough quantities of food protein, should fortify themselves against liver damage by adding protein (amino acids) to the diet in concentrated form.

Cirrhosis of the liver means an actual hardening of this vital organ. When this most serious of liver diseases sets in, the organ changes its sponge-like structure, since the tissues become fibrous and hard.

At first the organ enlarges, then gradually becomes harder and smaller, even shrinking so greatly in some instances that blood coming from the intestines laden with food elements cannot pass through the liver filter on its way to the heart.

As cirrhosis progresses, this blood stagnates in the veins of the abdomen, and the blood plasma seeps out of the blood vessels into the abdominal cavity. Heavy use of alcohol and cirrhosis go together. Cirrhosis of the liver, as well as ulcers of the stomach, is known as the "drunkard's disease."

The effect of alcohol upon liver tissues is bad enough, but since most heavy drinkers are also light eaters, the combination of too much alcohol plus too little protein is bound, in the long run, to damage the liver cells.

However, cirrhosis of the liver is not the exclusive "privilege" of alcoholics, for it has been observed recently that more than half the victims of this disease have never touched a drop of liquor in their lives!

This serious disease of the liver can occur solely through adherence to an unbalanced diet. Insufficient protein, as well as inadequate amounts of the vitamin B-complex group, may produce cirrhosis of the liver in the most abstemious of persons.

Once established, cirrhosis is a tricky disease, rarely curable. How-ever, if discovered and treated in its early stages, it can be arrested.

And since the liver has remarkable recuperative powers, it can resume nearly normal functioning while maintained in this arrested condition. However, a lapse into the old, unwise eating habits will bring back the cirrhosis to an even more severe degree.

Early symptoms of cirrhosis are vague, so that a definite diagnosis is hard to make until the disease is well advanced. But there are certain danger signals which should make anyone stop and look to make sure that the liver is being properly nourished with all the protein and vitamins it needs.

These danger signals are loss of appetite, a sense of fullness or discomfort after meals, nausea, constipation, loss of weight and a swollen abdomen. Certain amino acids, especially methionine and cysteine, as well as the vitamin choline have proved unusually efficient in treating cirrhosis of the liver.

When this treatment is also fortified by a diet low in fat but high in protein and natural carbohydrates such as whole grains and certain vegetables, the disease responds quickly.

A number of patients being treated with choline therapy showed distinct improvement within one week after this vitamin was first given. Particularly was it effective in the fatty type of liver degeneration.

When the liver is not functioning properly, it deposits fats, lipids they are called, within its cells, thereby lessening its own ability to perform efficiently. Choline is a valuable lipotropic (fat dissolving) factor. Even after a single meal with high fat content, choline has been observed to exert its fat-dissolving influence upon the liver.

Although small amounts of choline have a marked effect in preventing deposits of liver fat, larger amounts of concentrated choline (up to 1,000 milligrams daily) are necessary to make sure that the fat in the liver does not exceed its normal level.

Choline is a wonderful aid in promoting normal distribution of food fat throughout the body in its proper "depots," thereby preventing fatty accumulations in unwanted places, especially in the liver.

Choline is found in most high protein foods like red meat. It is also present in substantial amounts in the herb fenugreek. It might be a good idea for anyone predisposed to liver disorders to replace tea and coffee as a mealtime and between meal beverages with a tea made from this herb to assure adequate choline for the liver.

With the liver, that hard-working, most versatile of all the vital organs, the motto should be: "An ounce of mental and nutritional prevention is worth a pound cf medical cure!"

Chapter 9

Indigestion, Constipation, Ulcers and Colitis

One evening while delivering a lecture in Detroit, I was surprised to see a man in the fourth row get up and leave. It was not the fact of his leaving that surprised me. I knew that this particular man had come especially to learn more about the eccentricities of his intestinal tract, since he had been a victim of chronic constipation for years, and my lecture that night had the functioning of the digestive system for its subject.

The next day I happened to meet this same man on the street as I was leaving my hotel. Before I could greet him, he said, a bit testily, "You sure disappointed me last night. I made a special effort to get to that lecture because I thought you were going to talk about constipation, and then you changed it to 'indigestion.' "

"But constipation is the result of indigestion . . ," I started to explain. "Not with me," he interrupted. "I got swell digestion. It's just my darn bowels that are all haywire." Strange as it may seem, this man is not an isolated case in believing that indigestion and constipation are two widely divorced subjects.

From the hundreds of questions asked at my lectures, I find a widespread misconception that indigestion is an exclusive ailment of the stomach, while the evil of constipation lurks wholly within the intestinal tract.

The work of the intestines is so closely tied in to the entire digestive process that I consider indigestion and constipation an inseparable subject. Both are ailments of the digestive tract a tract that begins in the mouth and ends at the rectum.

More individuals suffer from discomforts, disorders and diseases arising within this tract than from any other single bodily function.

And when we stop to think that the digestive tract is not nothing more nor less than the human food factory, it becomes quite obvious that we, as a human mechanism, cannot operate at top efficiency when the processing plant where our food is received and prepared has slow-downs and break-downs.

The Human Food Factory

The human food factory has two jobs to do: First, it must break down the large food molecules into infinitely smaller molecules that can be transported throughout the body, to pass through the cell and tissue walls.

A starch molecule in that bite of wheat bread you ate for breakfast cannot possibly penetrate the intestinal wall into the bloodstream until it is reduced to the proper size molecule by digestion. In this process of digestion, starch molecules are broken down into sugars; fats and oils into soaps; proteins into amino acids.

Second, the human food factory must convert alien food molecules into specific human molecules. The food we put into our stomachs contains molecules of many kinds: cow's milk, chicken and animal flesh, fish oil, grain starch, vegetable fibers, and many others.

We swallow beef protein, for instance, but not one single tissue cell in the human body can be repaired and maintained by the protein in beef flesh, until this animal protein is transformed into molecules of human protein, that is, into amino acids which, in turn, are reconstructed by the body into human protein, the kind that is usable by our body cells.

Therefore, the food we take into our bodies is merely the raw material from which our

76

digestive tract processes and extracts the nutritive elements that actually feed our tissue, nerve and bone cells.

Every bite of food we put into our mouths is destined for the ultimate goal of these cells. It is not the stomach we feed we feed our cells! The flour that is rolled by the barrel into the bakeries is not the bread that goes on your table any more than the bite of bread you eat is the substance that feeds the body cells.

The flour (whole grain, of course, for white flour is a crime against digestion) must first be mixed with other ingredients and broken down by heat into "digestible" form before it emerges as a loaf of edible bread. In turn, the bite of bread we eat must be mixed with certain salivary secretions, digestive acids and enzymes before it, too, can be converted into "digestible" form for assimilation into the bloodstream where it is carried throughout the body to the eagerly awaiting cells.

The organs involved in the digestive processes are several and their ailments are more than several. When we speak of the "digestive apparatus" we generally mean the stomach, the duodenum, the small intestine, the large intestine or colon, the liver, the gall bladder and the pancreas, although this latter organ is also a member of the endocrine gland system.

There are many causes of indigestion, as well as its related maladies: constipation, ulcers and colitis. Symptoms of these disorders and diseases are many and varied. This is not surprising when we consider that the entire digestive function is a long, complicated, delicately balanced process; in fact, so delicately balanced is the digestive process that slight causes often throw it out of gear.

In addition to disorders of the digestive organs themselves, there are three basic reasons for indigestion and constipation: eating the wrong kind of food, eating too much and eating too quickly.

At least three-fourths of the American people eat far more food than is actually required to keep the body properly stoked with fuel.

Yet they are surprised when gas, sour stomach, belching, nausea and constipation, as well as numerous other signs of digestive upsets, indicate that the "food factory" is not operating up to its intended efficiency.

The common tendency is to blame the trouble on "something I ate." But, unless that something was too great a food atrocity, it alone did not cause the whole trouble. However, combined with other unwise foods, swallowed in improperly chewed hunks, washed down by gulps of liquid, plus generous gulps of air, it all can add up to indigestion trouble in the "food factory."

Gases from undigested, fermenting foods are absorbed from the alimentary tract; acids and wastes resulting from fermented food may poison the bloodstream, thereby upsetting the entire body, leading to almost any disorder, all the way from a feverish cold to a chronic condition like ulcerative colitis.

When I mentioned the basic reasons for digestive upsets, I purposely omitted one of the most flagrant offenders the mind. For years, medical science has known that strong emotions can upset the stomach.

Nearly every formal textbook on physiology stresses the fact that bad news or emotionally disturbing topics taken to the dinner table can make the stomach cease secreting the all-important digestive juices, allowing food to remain unprocessed for proper absorption through the intestinal walls, thus bringing on acute upsets such as nausea, vomiting, headache or abdominal cramping, to say nothing of constipation.

Many years ago a doctor had a patient with a stomach wound that would not heal. Through this deep fistula in the stomach wall, the doctor was able to observe the actual workings of the human stomach during the digestive process.

Especially was the doctor impressed with the discovery that when the patient was worried or angry, his stomach worked far less efficiently than when he was calm and relaxed.

Often such symptoms as fullness, swelling, nausea, belching, sour stomach, halitosis and diarrhea or constipation are the evidences of a disturbed mind. An old saying, "The stomach is the dumping ground for all worries," certainly had its basis in fact. At least 60 percent of the stomach disorders seen by physicians are diagnosed as "nervous indigestion."

Mental strain can make the appetite decrease and digestion slow down. An active imagination, coupled with emotionalism, can produce actual symptoms such as heartburn, distress, vomiting and tenderness in the otherwise normal stomach.

Certain worriers can actually cause their stomachs to dilate because of disturbed muscles in the stomach walls. Violent emotions such as hysteria and terror, as well as melancholy and intense mental strain, commonly bring on vomiting.

Worry and emotional strain can cause diarrhea, mucous colitis and constipation, because the upset mind disturbs the sensitive nervous mechanism that controls movement of the intestines. A famous physiologist once said: "In man, the same as in the other mammals, there is a direct nerve connection between the brain and the gut.

Any sudden, violent emotion reacts directly on the intestines, usually either causing them to empty suddenly, diarrhea, or tying them into such a knot that constipation is the result." A recent case history provides a good illustration of the row the mind can kick up in the digestive organs.

After a whirlwind courtship, Sally King married a handsome soldier in Boston, her home town. She had known him only three months. The honeymoon was only five days, and then Dick was sent overseas on active duty where he remained for nearly three years.

Finally Dick came back and was discharged. After a blissful reunion in the home of Sally's parents, the question of setting up housekeeping arose.

Sally was greatly taken aback when she learned that Dick had taken it for granted that she knew he was a farmer and intended to go back to the Indiana farm his father had waiting for him.

She insisted that she was a city girl and knew nothing about farming; Dick was equally insistent that he was a farmer and knew nothing about wage-earning. Dick won.

So in a somewhat strained atmosphere they began their married life in the bungalow Dick's father had built for them on a hundred acres of his own large farm. Dick's parents liked Sally and did everything they could to make her welcome.

She liked them, too, and tried to be happy in her new home. But the strangeness of the unaccustomed routines irritated and upset her; the animals frightened her; the country silence made her nervous. She kept silent about her discontentment, for she truly loved her husband and was determined not to show her unhappiness.

Before long, Sally was seized with violent abdominal pains. Dick rushed her off to Indianapolis where a clinical examination failed to disclose anything organically wrong with her. Oddly enough, her pain disappeared entirely while she was in the city.

Not long after returning to the farm, the pain returned with even greater intensity, this time coupled with alternating diarrhea and constipation. The local doctor pronounced it "colitis," gave her some powders, put her on a bland diet. But this treatment brought little relief from her acute abdominal symptoms.

In desperation, Dick suggested that Sally go home to Boston to consult her old family physician. Eagerly Sally accepted the suggestion, although she felt a little conscience-stricken at the station when Dick and his parents were so worried about her going all the way alone when she was "so sick."

To tell the truth, she was not sick at all as she got on the train; she felt fine, even elated at the prospect of leaving Indiana far behind for the streets of her beloved Boston.

Even then, on the train, Sally suspected the truth about her case as it later came out in the diagnosis given by her family doctor.

"Young lady," he said sternly, "there's nothing wrong with your colon. The trouble is all in your mind. You're fretting yourself into intestinal trouble for some reason or other, and the sooner you stop worrying about what can't be changed, the quicker you'll see this 'colitis' disappear."

Chronic fatigue is another case for much distress in the gastro-intestinal (digestive) tract. It reduces the body's nerve cell energy to so low a level that normal nervous stimulation is lacking when the digestive process has need of strong nerve impulses to start the digestive machinery in the human "food factory."

Many stubborn cases of indigestion and constipation clear up after the fatigue symptoms have been relieved. Dr. Walter Alvarez, the famous physician of the Mayo Clinic, said: "The commonest causes of 'nervous indigestion' are fatigue, worry, hypersensitiveness and insomnia."

Too many persons live by their emotions rather than by their reasoning powers. And the tensions caused by this type of emotionalism upset the balance of the chemical activity in the stomach, for the stomach is a veritable laboratory with its powerful acid digestive juices that break down solid food (protein especially) to a pulpy mass much as solid tree trunks are broken down by acids at the pulp mills to produce paper.

Mental tension and strain cause the adrenal glands (we met these two endocrine glands in the last chapter where they were causing high blood pressure) to shoot over secretions of that powerful "emergency hormone," adrenalin, into the blood.

It is believed that the real purpose of adrenalin in the blood is to have the effect of suspending digestive activity so that the heart can rush all possible blood to the part of the body that needs to react instantly in some crisis for instance, to the limbs when a supreme effort must be made to jump to safety from the path of a speeding automobile.

But when mental tension becomes habitual, the adrenal glands keep on sending adrenalin into the bloodstream when it is distinctly not wanted, with the result that the internal organs suffer, particularly the stomach, which fails to get the blood needed to maintain this laboratory of the "food factory" supplied with all the needed chemicals for good digestion.

My advice to any sufferer of indigestion or constipation is to make sure first that the trouble does not arise within the mind. Especially is this the case with persons who eat when overly tired or when agitated, or who eat alone, harassed by the thought of their loneliness.

In these latter instances, the mere presence of a pleasant companion to talk with at mealtimes often causes the symptoms of indigestion to clear up entirely. Mealtime was meant to be a period of enjoyment and relaxation; why endanger the health of the entire body by taking our troubles to the table with us? A little cheer and less self-pity will work wonders with many cases of "nervous indigestion."

Chapter 9

Stomach Indigestion and Ulcers

The stomach is a bottle-shaped bag, with a volume of about 61 cubic inches, lying somewhat crosswise in the upper part of the abdomen, the larger end turned toward the left. It consists of three firmly united layers: the external peritoneal, or membranous, covering; the middle layer of muscles; and the delicate inner mucous membrane lining.

At either end of this "bottle" is a powerful circular muscle that contracts to keep the stomach passageway closed except at the moments when food is either entering the stomach or passing out of it into the duodenum (the upper part of the small intestine and sometimes called the second stomach). The upper entrance to the stomach is called the cardia, and the lower exit is the pylorus.

Both these muscular "doorways" into the stomach will open only when conditions are right. In the case of the cardia, it takes a delicate stimulus such as that exerted by thoroughly masticated food.

If a coarse, solid object such as a bite of improperly chewed food strikes the cardia, it closes all the tighter, refusing the food hunk entrance to the stomach where a solid mass might damage the delicate stomach lining. This creates an unpleasant sensation of pressure within the upper abdomen.

So, you see a good part of your sensations of indigestion can arise from bites of poorly chewed food lying in the esophagus (tube leading from the throat to the cardia) rather than in the stomach itself.

Those of you who have heard me lecture know that I am strongly opposed to the American habit of soft-drink imbibing. This is one reason why: The cardia, being a faithful watchman, also tries to prevent any biting, stinging or caustic fluid from entering the stomach where it could injure that delicate membranous wall.

Therefore, when carbonated water, beer, too is taken, it collects in a pool above the stomach, creating pressure not only because of its weight, but also because of the high degree of gas it contains.

Finally, after enough gas has been belched up to reduce the stinging feel of the carbonated pool, the cardia will open. In view of the needless discomfort carbonated beverages can cause to a person already suffering from an impaired digestive apparatus, it is sheer folly to multiply the misery by imbibing fluids that are nothing but a distressing habit.

When the stomach is healthy, its walls possess a muscular tension that makes them elastic. This elasticity prevents the stomach from sagging under the weight of a meal.

But when this muscular tension has been decreased, either through disease or abuse, the stomach, when full, actually sags like a deflated balloon, hanging down into the pelvic area. On the other hand, a healthy stomach receiving food will expand gradually, like a balloon, without altering its original shape.

Of course, a sagging, pendulant stomach is incapable of performing a good job of digestion. Food remains in it too long, and the pressure of this filled sack is felt against the other organs.

When food enters the stomach, the glands in the wall begin pouring out their digestive juices. These juices are acid; they have to be acid to break down and dissolve the tough food fibers.

Therefore, anyone who swallows continual doses of widely advertised "alkalizers" to "relieve" indigestion is merely adding fuel to the flame of his digestive troubles.

Nine times out of ten and particularly in older persons what is needed in cases of true indigestion is more stomach acid, not less. And to decrease what little acid there is by neutralizing it with repeated doses of an alkali is to defeat the very purpose for which the remedy is taken.

If the chemistry of the stomach juices were more widely understood, the manufacturers of these useless even harmful digestive remedies would have to find some other product to publicize.

What happens to the food after it reaches the stomach makes an interesting story. Contrary to popular belief, the food does not lay any which way in the stomach; it is neatly arranged in definite layers.

The first food to arrive is deposited next to the stomach wall; the subsequent batches are piled in layers upon the first, something like a layer cake, so that the last food eaten lies toward the center. This, by the way, is why an autopsy made in crime detection can tell quite accurately the hour of death from the contents of the stomach.

The stomach does not lie quiet during this process of digestion as it does when empty. The moment food arrives sometimes even before, when the thought and sight of appetizing food starts the digestive juices flowing the floor of the stomach begins to move in waves.

Someone has described this motion as resembling the waves a photographer produces in a pan of developing solution in order to achieve the highest degree of chemical action on the film. And that, exactly, is the purpose of this stomach motion or peristalsis to mix the semi-solid food mass with the stomach acids.

When the layer of food lying next to the stomach wall has been thoroughly churned around and mixed with the gastric acids, it flows to the deepest part of the stomach "bottle" near which is located the pylorus, or exit.

Remember this, for it is very important: The pylorus normally remains closed and opens only under certain conditions. Unless the food mass that comes into the neighborhood of the pylorus is properly acid, the pylorus remains closed, for it is supposed to admit acidized masses only into the duodenum, or upper intestine.

If the food mass is thoroughly mixed with the acid gastric juices, the pylorus will open and permit a small portion to pass into the small intestine.

The instant that the mass touches the alkaline mucous membrane lining of the small intestine, the pylorus closes again, opening only when the alkaline digestive secretions of the duodenum have thoroughly treated the first batch that passed through.

And so on, until the entire contents of the stomach have been reduced to a properly acidized mass and then emptied into the small intestine for further digesting.

Dr. Kahn, the eminent European physiologist, compares the pylorus to a railway switch that allows only a certain amount of rail traffic to pass at specific times.

This opening and shutting of the pylorus goes on for several hours, until all the acidized mass has been passed from the stomach into the small intestine.

So delicately poised is the nervous mechanism of the pylorus that this process of emptying the stomach is easily upset by the wrong kind of food, by improper acidity of the gastric juices, by strong medicine, or by emotion. Strenuous physical activity that produces heavy fatigue also prevents the digestive mechanism from responding in a normal manner to this necessary process of emptying.

When, for any of these reasons, emptying the stomach does not take place on schedule, it is because the pyloric muscle at this opening between the stomach and the duodenum refuses to contract sufficiently to allow the passage of food masses.

Thereupon, the half-digested food remains too long in the stomach, causing indigestion with its many distressing symptoms. Ulcers are the most frequently encountered malady of the stomach. What causes these open sores to break out in the lining of the stomach?

You will remember that the digestive juices secreted by glands in the stomach wall must be acid to break down and digest even the toughest piece of meat. But what about the stomach wall? It is flesh, and certainly more susceptible to acid than a piece of animal muscle! So what is to keep the gastric acids from digesting the stomach itself?

Under normal circumstances, the stomach secretes substances that form a protective coating over the entire membranous wall for the very purpose of preventing the gastric acids from attacking the walls of this organ.

In other words, these protective substances flow over and seal the tender mucous membrane lining against attack from acid digestive juices.

However, since the production and secretion of all glandular fluids are largely affected by the nervous system, a series cf emotional tensions can so lower the power of the stomach to produce these protective substances that the gastric acids actually do find a poorly coated spot in the membrane lining of the stomach and begin attempting to break it down! After repeated attacks, the membrane is weakened and an open sore results.

This sore is the ulcer. At first the ulcer may be no larger than a pinpoint, but if allowed to continue unhealed, the wound grows to the size of a dime, in serious cases even to the size of a half dollar.

The ladies may be interested to learn that up until a decade or so ago when the feminine form was encircled by tightly fitting corsets, the women had four to five times as many stomach ulcers as men. But today men become easier victims of ulcers in the stomach wall, as well as those sores that occur in the duodenum.

The tight, waist-pinching corset that was a necessity in the wardrobe of every well-dressed, "decent" woman back in grandmother's day exerted so much pressure on the stomach and the intestines that the entire digestive function was seriously impeded.

Ulcers were the result. But when fashion turned sensible for a change and allowed the American woman to retain her natural form instead of squeezing her organs to achieve the barbaric "wasp waist," female ulcer victims became fewer and fewer.

In view of this, I hope that no sensible woman will allow herself to be corseted into ulcers by any future fashion edicts that may emanate from Paris or Hollywood. Worry and irritating foods, however, are now the prime causes of gastric ulcers. This is so axiomatic that certain persons are referred to as "the ulcer type."

Usually they are business or professional men, living under the constant strain of trying to be, or continuing to be, successful. Or they may be individuals, whose ambition for success or recognition has been frustrated, bringing on a constant feeling of defeat.

A great deal of research has been done to find not only a cure, but a preventive as well, against the formation of these ulcers in the digestive tract. Ever so often the news columns will carry a story of some highly touted drug discovery that it is hoped will eliminate the prevalence of this "civilized" disease. Sometimes these new drugs work, and again they do not; even though they may bring some relief from the pain of ulcers, they often cause allergies or other digestive upsets.

News that Russian medical men were treating stomach ulcers with honey looks particularly promising, since it involves a natural substance instead of a strong drug.

The patients were given about 250 grams of honey a day for periods of from fourteen to eighteen days. Many of the patients reported that all pain disappeared after the first day.

Honey, of course, is a pre-digested food and it seems logical that it could play an effective part in correcting the poor digestive functioning that leads to ulcers. Recent tests conducted by Dr. Cheney at the Stanford University School of Medicine on laboratory animals would indicate that a diet rich in "vitamin U" reduces the tendency toward stomach ulcers. This "vitamin U" is found in raw foods.

Although there is no proof that the stomach of a guinea pig behaves exactly like that of a human being, Dr. Cheney believes that more raw foods in the diet would be advisable for ulcer patients.

The raw foods that he recommends be included in the diet in generous quantities (provided there is no other intolerance to them) are: kale, lettuce, cabbage, fresh greens, raw egg yolk, soybean oil, olive oil and liver fat. Dr. Cheney advances the theory that the number of gastric ulcers is increasing because we eat far too few raw, unheated foods, thereby losing the "vitamin U" which is destroyed by heat.

To date one of the most successful treatments for ulcers of the stomach has been obtained with amino acids. This is logical because amino acids are nothing more than food protein broken down into the form in which the human cells can utilize the protein food eaten.

This conversion of protein foods into amino acids is a regular part of every digestive performance. However, research has made it possible to produce amino acids outside the body, in concentrated form.

Since protein, in the form of amino acids, is the natural material the body uses to build and repair tissue, treating damaged stomach tissue with amino acids is a sensible repair job.

Astonishing work with this amino acid treatment for ulcers has been done by Dr. Co Tui, brilliant Chinese research scientist at New York University. In order to prepare four patients with severely ulcerated stomachs for the operating table, they were fed concentrated doses of amino acids.

The patients selected were indigents from Bellevue Hospital whose chances of coming off the operating table alive were slight. These wretched ulcer victims were desperately in need of the new tissues, the new resistance that the amino acids could give them.

Amino acids were given the four patients every two hours. Within 24 hours the gnawing pain that characterizes ulcers had disappeared. And 96 hours after the treatment was started, all internal bleeding had been checked.

The patients began to show external signs of improvement; their skin took on a healthier color, and their flabby muscles began to strengthen. Ten days from the first dose of amino acids, each patient had gained from seven to ten pounds.

One of the patients demanded his clothes and went home; he said if he could get that much better in only 10 days by such simple treatment, he saw no sense in surgery. The other three patients, however, submitted to the surgeon's knife.

Ironically, in one case the ulcer was found to be healed over completely and this took place in only ten days after the treatment with amino acids was started! In the other two cases, the ulcers had already started satisfactory healing. Given a few more days of amino acid treatment, the operations could have been cancelled.

Dr. Co Tui was so encouraged by this first experiment that he later selected another group of 27 patients whose ulcers dated all the way from one month to twenty years.

In every case, the acute pain that characterizes peptic ulcer disappeared within 48 hours after the first feeding of amino acids was given. The healing process was watched by X-ray; gradually the ulcer craters were observed to fill up with new, healthy tissue that had been stimulated by the amino acids.

In not one of these 27 cases of stomach ulcer was surgery necessary; every patient's ulcer, regardless of its severity, healed by itself under the stimulus of the new tissue provided and nourished by the amino acids.

Amino acids are not claimed as a "cure" for ulcers. Instead, they are the food that can build the new tissue necessary to fill in the raw crater-like sores made in the stomach lining. An ulcer is nothing more than a breakdown in healthy tissue.

Amino acids can heal ulcers without danger of injuring any other of the delicate digestive mechanisms. But the development of another ulcer from the same cause as the first one is something the patient must take care does not happen again.

The wise course for any victim of stomach ulcers to follow is to set about healing the present sore by some safe, proved means; and then to ascertain with as much certainty as possible the exact cause for the ulcer to avoid a recurrence of this needless ailment. Especially is this a sane course to follow, if you are the "ulcer type."

Intestines Constipation and Colitis

The intestines or bowels are divided into two sections; the small intestine which includes the upper section, known as the duodenum, and the large bowel, known as the colon. Food undergoing the digestive process passes from the stomach directly into the duodenum (so named because it is 12 finger lengths long). Here the pancreas and liver (the latter through the gall bladder) and their secretions do the job of digestion.

The food mass then passes through each of the numerous loops of the small intestine, all the while becoming more and more "digested." Then, after the nutritive elements are absorbed from it, the mass is pushed along into the colon where it travels down to the rectum and out of the body.

The motion that keeps this food mass from stagnating in the intestines is also called peristalsis, and its movements resemble the wave-like, nervous contractions that take place in the stomach to assure proper mixing of the food with the gastric juices.

The prime factor that contributes to chronic constipation is a slowing down of this peristaltic movement.

Here in the intestinal "department" of the human food factory the digestive processing is completed, and the "shipping" begins. This "shipping" of the body's nourishment to its consumers the cells takes place via the walls of the small intestine directly into the bloodstream.

Fixed to the walls of the small intestine are millions upon millions of small nipple-like organs called villi. They work like suction pumps, taking up portions of the now semi-liquid food mass, extracting the wanted nutritive elements, filtering them into the bloodstream, and rejecting the waste matter.

This process of pumping nourishment from the food in the intestinal tract into the bloodstream is called assimilation. When a person is said to have "poor assimilation," it means that for one reason or another only a negligible portion of the nutritive elements in the food mass gets through these villi into the bloodstream.

Hence not enough nourishment reaches the body cells, and they suffer from malnutrition. In other words, a breakdown in assimilation takes place when the food products of the human food factory remain in the factory instead of being shipped out to the cell consumers.

Many persons whose diet is both sane and adequate are nevertheless victims of poor assimilation all because the villi in the small intestine cannot assimilate the food for lack of which the body cells are starving.

Poor assimilation can be caused by food that is inadequately digested by the time it reaches the duodenum, since not enough fluids have been provided by the various digestive organs. Or, more commonly, poor assimilation is the result of a mucus-clogged intestinal wall.

If abnormal quantities of stagnant mucus are allowed to gather and thicken in these villi suction-pumps, naturally they cannot work efficiently. And when the villi pumps are slowed down, or put out of operation in large numbers because of mucus plugs, the body cells are bound to go hungry.

When a cell dies of starvation, there is trouble ahead for the organism where those cells are located! That, in brief, is the beginning of all disease and degeneration starving and dying cells.

The obvious action called for when assimilation cannot take place because of clogged villi is to find something that will remove the mucus plugs from them, restoring them to full operation. In a previous chapter I mentioned an herb called fenugreek which has the peculiar ability to dissolve stagnant mucus.

Numerous victims of constipation and poor assimilation have reported to me that they overcame these disorders to a large degree after cleansing the excess mucus from their intestinal tracts by regular use of a tea made from the herb fenugreek.

Constipation is an ailment afflicting everyone at some time or other throughout a lifetime. This is true because constipation is actually the result of a digestive upset, and rare indeed is the person who, at one time or another, has not had his digestion interrupted and slowed down for some cause.

When the exit from the stomach the pylorus refuses to open, allowing food masses to remain too long in the stomach, the entire operation of the intestinal tract is likewise upset. Constipation is the result of this behind-schedule lag.

Therefore, constipation actually begins in the stomach with impaired digestion. Consequently, constipation cannot be cured by the habitual use of cathartics or enemas. In going about the intelligent correction of chronic constipation, the first step is to attempt to speed up digestion.

It has been estimated that 99 out of 100 victims of chronic constipation also suffer from subnormal digestive functioning. In other words, the human food factory is slowed down to such an extent during the early processing that the later work of assimilation and elimination are thrown off schedule.

The stomach "department" of this human food factory quite often falls down on the job, not only because of weakly acid digestive juices, but also because some of its enzymes do not show up in sufficient numbers to keep production at top speed.

Enzymes are essential workers, being complex substances produced by both plants and animals. In humans, enzymes present in digestive juices have a specific task of speeding up the course of certain chemical reactions vital to good digestion.

Therefore, digestion usually proceeds according to schedule when the correct proportions of the various digestive enzymes are present in the human food factory. These enzymes attack the food mass like a flock of chickens devouring corn.

Each enzyme attacks a particular type of food, either protein; carbohydrate or fat; when the enzyme needed to speed up digestion of one or more of these food types is not present in sufficient quantities that food is found to be "hard to digest."

Enzymes are found in secretions from glands of the mouth, the pancreas, the stomach, and the intestines. Science has found that papain, an enzyme extracted from a tropical fruit called the papaya, is an effective stimulator of enzymatic action in human digestion.

Because sufficient enzymes are vital to good digestion, the very first step toward avoiding constipation is to make sure that the food being digested is supplied with enough of these digestive "speeder-uppers."

This can be done ordinarily by building up the general health through sane living and proper diet, and by stimulating the secretion of body enzymes through supplying papain to the digestive tract. Stubborn cases of constipation have been known to yield to the added stimulus of the papaya enzyme.

Because going to stool is largely a matter of training and habit, persons who are thrown out of their regular routine often find them-selves the uncomfortable victims of constipation. Especially does this occur when traveling? Individuals who otherwise are almost complete strangers to the misery of constipation will find themselves confronted with the unyielding problem of a stubborn bowel when on vacation, or on a long trip.

Different hours of waking or eating are sometimes enough to upset the temperamental intestinal processes, or it may be that the diet while away from home is too rich or too abundant.

Then there are the persons who suddenly find themselves forced into a sedentary life after having enjoyed an active, outdoor life for many years. The bowels are usually the first part of the body to show their resentment of this change.

Certain occupations, too, such as operators of public vehicles or other employment where the duties of the job come before personal comfort all contribute to constipation.

From my personal contact with thousands of health students, I have long realized the prevalence and the seriousness of the constipation problem. The ideal way, of course, to conquer constipation is through making the digestive process more efficient and by acquiring proper living and eating habits. These are the methods I have taught by lecture and by book for a number of years.

I could only wish that all who have heard my lectures or who have read my books would profit by this sane program for overcoming constipation. But the fact that many of them do not so profit is made all too evident to me by the nature of the questions that are asked at my lectures. Constipation continues to be the number one health problem.

This is true, perhaps, because we cannot turn back the tide of modern living too little exercise, not enough food with natural vitamins and minerals, and too much nervous tension. Especially is the mind a serious factor in this problem of conquering constipation.

If everyone could be assured that no emotional crisis would ever arise to upset the digestion, then constipation would not be as prevalent an ailment as it is today.

Or if they could be promised that no break in their daily routine would disturb the schedule of bowel evacuation, constipation might fade into the background of common disorders. But no such assurance is forthcoming, and constipation continues to be the personal, everyday concern of millions of persons.

Obviously some safe, natural remedy must be provided for the victims of occasional constipation. Mineral oil once widely advertised and used as a "safe" laxative has been proved harmful since it irritates the intestinal wall and interferes with proper absorption of certain vitamins.

Moreover, some of the oil is absorbed into the bloodstream, thereby creating a potentially dangerous situation. What about the breakfast foods guaranteed to add "bulk" to the diet? Most of these, particularly whole bran, are highly irritating to a sensitive bowel and should never be resorted to as a remedy for constipation.

Anyone who has ever heard me lecture, or who follows the health regimen I advocate, knows that I am violently opposed to harsh laxatives, cathartics and purgatives because they are inestimably injurious to the gastro-intestinal tract.

Yet, because the problem of constipation continues to harass thousands of persons every day, we must be practical about this matter of intestinal elimination.

When in a health dilemma, the best recourse is to Nature. In her wisdom and beneficence she has provided in the forests and fields the natural substances that can be taken into the body without causing injury to the delicate digestive tract.

After careful experimentation, I have found that six natural substances may safely be used as a mild bowel activator when the absolute need for a laxative arises. This does not mean that I condone the lazy habit of depending upon artificial methods to accomplish what should be done according to natural rhythm.

But, if and when the need arises for a safe treatment for constipation, ' remedies containing these six laxative herbs can be relied upon to act without injuring the bowel membranes or without becoming habit-forming, since they are natural substances: cascara sagrada; podophyllin extracted from mandrake root; alone obtained from aloes; ipecac; rhubarb root and licorice.

All six of these are plant substances, and do not approach the violence of synthetic compounds. Their action is natural and soothing.

For instance, the United States Dispensatory has this to say about rhubarb root as a laxative: "Because the movements of the upper bowel are not much affected, these drugs (rhubarb) are incapable of violent purgation, and for the same reason are less likely to produce secondary constipation than those drugs which empty the upper bowel."

Therefore, being practical about a health problem that seems to increase rather than improve, if constipation resists conscientious treatment by diet and exercise, the next best method is the occasional use of a remedy containing these natural, stimulating herbal substances.

This brings up the ever-present question: "How can I tell when I am constipated?" On the average, a bowel movement once every twenty four hours is sufficient, although there are persons who go to stool several times a day, and still others experience no discomfort from a bowel movement only once in every two or three days.

Therefore, the question is not so much how often, but how much fecal mass remains in the intestinal tract for an unnecessary length of time.

In a healthy colon, about four-fifths of the fecal matter to be evacuated should be present in the rectum when the person goes to stool, so that after a complete movement, only about one-fifth of the intestinal waste should remain behind in the upper sections of the intestine.

For that reason, constipation may occur regardless of the number of movements, if considerable quantities of waste material remain in the large intestine after evacuation. It is well known to physicians treating intestinal ailments that a patient can have a bowel movement daily and yet be constipated, simply because as much or more matter remains in the upper section of the colon than was evacuated.

A normal stool, evacuated at the proper time, should have the form of a column; if it is too hard, so that, instead of a column, it comes out in small or ball-shaped pieces, then elimination is delayed, meaning that the bowel is constipated.

Constipation, in itself, is an unpleasant ailment and one that should never be allowed to continue any longer than it can be relieved. The seriousness of constipation goes even beyond this, for it is a potential threat to many of the graver diseases such as heart disorders, high blood pressure and diseases of the sexual organs.

Therefore, as you value your health, and physical and mental wellbeing, do not allow the insidious habit of constipation to fasten upon your intestinal tract!

Colitis is another ailment of the intestinal tract from which an untold number of victims suffer. Perhaps because of the deleterious effect a tense mind has on the entire digestive system, colitis is on the increase.

Especially is it a "white collar" disease, afflicting those engaged in sedentary occupations. Colitis is rarely found among persons performing heavy work. Women are the more susceptible sex, perhaps because of their more highly keyed nervous systems.

Colitis is found to develop between the ages of twenty and forty, as a general rule, and the most common symptoms are colicky pains in the abdomen, diarrhea alternating with constipation, as well as headaches in the forehead and at the back of the head.

To say "colitis" and expect to find the cause is like trying to locate a specific ailment by giving the symptom as "headache."

In fact, colitis might be called the "headache of the large bowel," since it is a disorder that arises from any one or more of various causes, none of which is readily located. However, the causes most often tagged are irritation in the bowel caused by parasites or bacteria, certain food allergies, and emotional strain.

Colitis is also divided into two kinds: mucous or spastic, and ulcerative. In the first type, because the lining of the large bowel is attacked, it secretes excess mucus, and often constricts so that the waste mass has great difficulty passing through on its way to the rectum.

Sometimes a bowel will be attacked by ulcers on the inner wall, leading to the more serious ulcerative colitis which demands drastic treatment immediately, since the ulcers may develop into a cancerous condition. In spastic colitis the main difficulty seems to arise from irregular, unpredictable upsets in the muscles controlling the contraction of the bowel.

Something, more often than not a mental stimulus, causes the bowel to squeeze together in some places and to remain relaxed in others.

This causes undue retention of waste matter, giving rise to the gas that produces the colicky pains characteristic of this ailment. Aside from the need to relax and obtain plenty of mild outdoor exercise, there are dietary means of treating colitis. Vitamins A and B-complex are unusually effective in treating disorders of the gastro-intestinal tract.

Especially vitamin A, since it strengthens the mucous membrane of the intestinal walls. The thiamin in B-complex, of course, feeds the intestinal nerves and helps induce better nervous control, both in the central nervous system and in the bowel.

In cases of ulcerative colitis, some successful treatments have been undertaken with amino acids on the same basis as the treatments given for ulcers of the stomach.

A bland diet is always best in treating any case of colitis that hangs on indefinitely. Foods should be soft and well cooked. Sour milk products or lactic acid capsules often prove soothing to an irritated colon, as well as providing an effective crusading force against undesirable bacteria in the colon.

Along with diet and dietary supplements should go outdoor exercise that stops short of fatigue, since exhaustion makes colitis worse. But probably as important as any other therapeutic measure is the need to relax, to stop worrying the colon by making it the chief topic of thought and conversation.

Plenty of rest and relaxing recreation will help build up the nervous stability needed to calm a spastic colon, as well as one that is ulcerated.

No discussion of the colon would be complete without mentioning that abused appendage, the vermiform appendix. No doubt you have heard it called a "biological mistake" that serves no purpose in the body, and, like the wisdom teeth, "the sooner out the better." Medical men who should know better are often guilty of making this dangerously erroneous remark about the appendix.

There is good and sufficient reason for every part, both large and small, of the entire human body. Many persons who have gotten rid of their "biological mistake" by having their appendix removed have later realized that they never felt quite the same!

Certainly their general health did not improve after divorcing themselves from their appendix. Many of them begin to experience chronic constipation, adhesions and other gastro-intestinal difficulties.

Contrary to the widely held medical opinion that the appendix serves no constructive purpose within the human body, it does have an important function that of lubricating the colon.

And, also contrary to popular belief, it is not the appendix that bothers you it is you who bother your appendix by allowing stagnant mucus and waste matter to accumulate in the cecum (the lower end of the ascending colon where the appendix is located).

Such an unhealthy accumulation is a certain cause of irritation: gradually the appendix will be affected, causing it to become clogged with foreign matter that has no chance of escaping, since the appendix is a sac with a one-way entrance. When this happens, the matter putrefies and irritation causes pus to form.

As long as the appendix is kept clean, it will be the best-behaved organ in the human body. But when it begins to fill up with pus, watch out! One fine day the appendix will become so inflamed, so distended that it will burst, spilling all that pus and poisonous stagnated mucus into the abdominal cavity.

When that happens, the terrifying verdict "peritonitis" may be heard; from then on it is anybody's guess how long the patient will survive. By this time, of course, it is much too late to take preventive measures to see that the appendix does not become clogged with waste matter that backs up from the cecum.

But a little forethought as to the predicament of the appendix when subjected to heavy modern meals, coupled with inadequate exercise, would have spared a lot of suffering.

114

Measures taken to keep the intestines reasonably free of excess mucus and to prevent waste matter from hanging around long enough to putrefy will help your appendix.

All in all, the human food factory is a pretty efficient operation. Particularly is this true, despite the abuse it receives. Yet the entire digestive operation is never any stronger than its weakest link; the gastrointestinal system should be spared irritation by both the mind and unwise diet and overwork.

Even the machines in a large factory are given time off for repairs. But we work our food processing machinery every day throughout the year without giving it a chance to rest.

That is why I long ago adopted a health measure for myself to which I attribute a large part of the fact that indigestion and constipation are disorders I write and talk about but never experience!

If you are seriously interested in keeping your digestive organs functioning healthily now and in later years, here is my sincere advice to you: Give the digestive mechanism an occasional "Sabbath" for resting.

I say occasional, although I would like to advocate resting your digestion every Sunday throughout the year; such a program would bring almost phenomenal results. But, as Charles F.

Kettering, vice president of General Motors, has said,

"if a proposal assumes any change in human nature, it won't work." I have learned that people prefer to sin, and then atone later for their sins. This is as true of their stomachs as it is of their souls.

Therefore, if you do not want my first-best advice to rest your stomach once a week, then here is my second-best suggestion: Spend one Sunday as usual, eating as you please; follow this day of indulgence by a Sunday of strict adherence to my Purifying Diet, given below.

During this day in which nothing but fruit juices and an herb tea (preferably made of fenugreek) enter the system, the stomach, intestines, colon, liver, kidneys will all have a chance to rest; at the same time, the body will receive nourishment with a minimum of effort for these organs.

The Purifying Diet

Night before: 2 herbal laxative tablets
Upon arising: I had a Glass of distilled water with one lemon juice

- 8AM.: Large glass of citrus juice
- 9AM.: Cup of herb tea made with fenugreek seeds

- 10AM.: Large glass of pineapple juice
- 11AM.: As much distilled water as you can comfortably drink
- 12Noon: Large glass of grape or apple juice
- 1PM.: Cup of herb tea made with fenugreek seeds
- 2PM.: Large glass of citrus juice
- 3P.M.: As much distilled water as you can comfortably drink
- 4PM.: Large glass of pineapple juice
- 5PM.: Cup of herb tea made with fenugreek seeds
- 6PM.: Large glass of grape or apple juice
- 7P.M.: As much distilled water as you can comfortably drink
- 8 PM.: Large glass of citrus juice
- 9PM.: Cup of herb tea made with fenugreek seeds
- 1OP.M.: 2 herbal laxative tablets

While it is true that 52 days of rest a year for the digestive tract would do twice as much good, still 26 days of abstinence from solid foods will bring proportionately beneficial results in a very short time.

I defy anyone to give the Purifying Diet a fair trial without finding himself feeling 100 percent more alive and vigorous within 60 days. The body will be stronger, the mind more alert, because you will be freed of accumulated toxins which cause sluggishness, torpidity of mind and body, biliousness, transient headaches.

Do not cheat, and make certain to follow the Purifying Diet on a non-working day when the body and mind are relaxing from the strain of a normal day's routine.

Besides giving your stomach a vacation once every fortnight, the Purifying Diet will accomplish another good for your body. It will help rescue you from that state of semi-dehydration in which a majority of persons keep their bodies at all times.

Most of us do not drink enough water. A man weighing 150 pounds is almost three fourths water; the blood is about 80 percent water; muscles are 75 to 80 percent water; and 85 percent of the gray matter of the brain is water.

All life processes start in water and must be continued in water. Water helps cleanse and flush impurities from the body. To neglect regular water drinking between meals is to leave the body wide open to many infections, some of them fatal.

Make it a faithfully followed habit to drink at least six glasses of pure water daily, unless otherwise directed by a competent physician. Drink more water if you so desire, but never less than six glasses in your waking hours.

If we expect our human food factory to pay health dividends, we must give it plenty of capital in the form of good food, rest, relaxation, and mental control. Don't make this vital mechanism

the dumping ground for all the mind's woes and
the appetite's caprices!

www.ingramcontent.com/pod-product-compliance
Lightning Source LLC
Chambersburg PA
CBHW060412290526
45791CB00002B/718